BACK AND HI

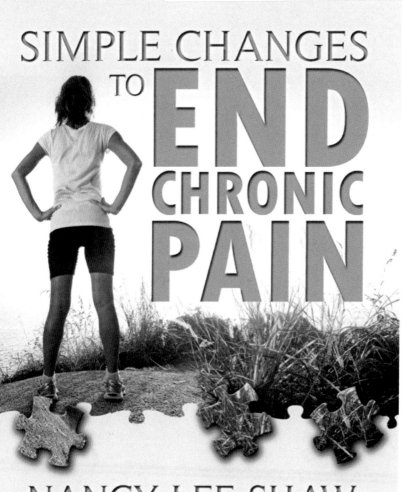

SIMPLE CHANGES TO END CHRONIC PAIN

NANCY LEE SHAW

Copyright © 2014 by Nancy Lee Shaw, M.S., M.A., MTPT
ISBN- 9781499159493
ISBN- 1499159498

All rights reserved. No part of this publication may be reproduced or transmitted in any form or by any means, electronic or mechanical, now known or thereafter invented, including photocopy, recording, computer scanning, or any information and retrieval system without the express written permission of Nancy Lee Shaw except in the case of brief quotations embodied in critical articles or reviews.

This publication is written and published to provide accurate and authoritative information in regard to the subject matter covered. It is published and sold with the understanding that the author, publisher, editors, and distributors are not engaged in rendering legal, medical, or other professional services. If medical or other expert assistance is required, the services of a competent professional person should be sought.

Notice: Reproduction is limited to the copyright restrictions listed above. For permission requests, contact Nancy Lee Shaw LLC at *myoconsult@verizon.net*

Editor: Anne DeMarsay, Voices Into Print
Book Design and Production: Dash Parham
Cover Design: Glendon Haddix, Streetlight Graphics
Illustrations: Keala Weinstock
Muscle Renderings: Dixie Vereen
Printed in the United States of America

www.createspace.com

Notes

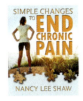 Be sure you refer to the parent book, *Simple Changes to End Chronic Pain,* for a full understanding of this booklet. Available at amazon.com

Myofascial Pain Treatment Center
Nancy L. Shaw, Director
6417 Loisdale Rd., Suite 308
Springfield, VA 22150
(703) 922-8250
myoconsult@verizon.net
http://nancyshawclinicandinstitute.com

 http://facebook.com/nancyshaw.56829

 http://linkedin.com/in/shawpainclinic

http://twitter.com/shawpainclinic

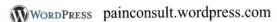 painconsult.wordpress.com

BACK PAIN

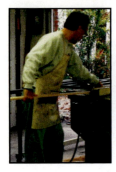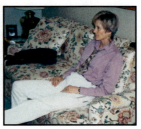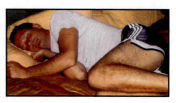

Back pain from these muscles in the **front of the body!**

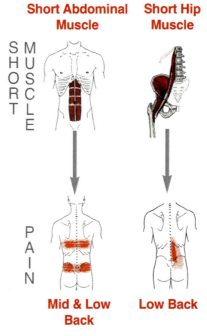

When you shorten these muscles as you lean forward, slouch, or curl, over time you will experience back pain.

Everyone knows that muscles do whatever you teach them to do. It is medically documented that continuously shortened muscles elicit pain in areas away from where they are located. Shortening muscles teaches them to stay short, resulting in pain.

It will hurt to stand upright until the muscles in the front are stretched and are taught to be elongated.

Back Pain

What do you usually do to lessen back pain?
You try to stretch the back: bending forward, bringing knees to chest, curling up to sleep, and sitting slouched. These actions feel good because they keep the muscles short, even when you are resting. Pain results when you try to stand upright and the muscles are pulled beyond their learned, short pattern of movement.

What should you do to eliminate back pain?
Change your standing, sitting, and sleeping postures as shown below, trying to position the body in a straight line.

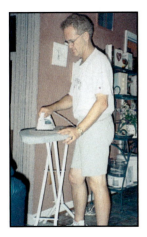
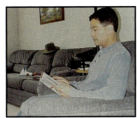
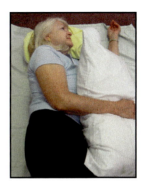

Additional information is included in *Simple Changes to End Chronic Pain.*

Back Pain

Note: Any time you sit, stand, or sleep with the body rounded forward or bent forward repeatedly, you shorten the very muscles that can result in *back pain*.

The critical point of understanding persistent, irritating, chronic **back pain** is to recognize that most of this pain is referred pain from the *two muscles* in the *front of the body* that are shown on the previous pages.

Yes, back pain that comes from muscles in the front of the body.
- Remember, muscles do whatever you do repeatedly that teaches them how to function. Think about it: all day you are leaning or bending forward, brushing teeth, putting shoes on, eating, sitting at a computer, leaning over the kitchen counter, slouching in a chair, curled sleeping, or driving; and the list goes on.

- How often do you bend backward or even stand upright for very long without slouching or bending forward? Not too often, if at all.

When you see people with back pain, they are often standing bent forward, holding their backs. It hurts to stand upright because the two muscles *in front* are too tight to let them stand up straight.

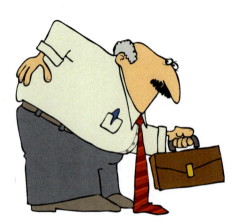

BACK PAIN

- Stretch the two front muscles by moving them backward with a standing or knee lunge, chest stretch, and end-of-bed stretch to decrease pain and to teach the muscles a new elongated habit of movement.

Grasp this one concept: back pain across the back and up and down the low back results from the two muscles indicated in the front of the body.

The following stretches are necessary to teach the muscles to move to a neutral, more elongated position than the short one that is resulting in back pain.

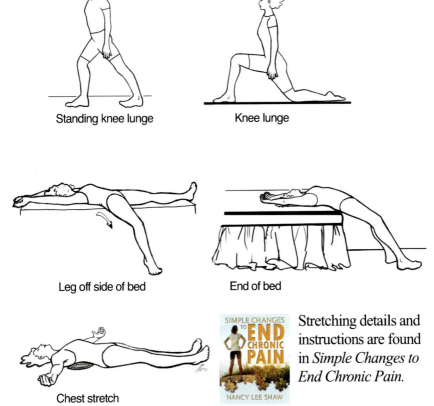

Standing knee lunge   Knee lunge

Leg off side of bed   End of bed

Chest stretch

Stretching details and instructions are found in *Simple Changes to End Chronic Pain.*

BACK PAIN

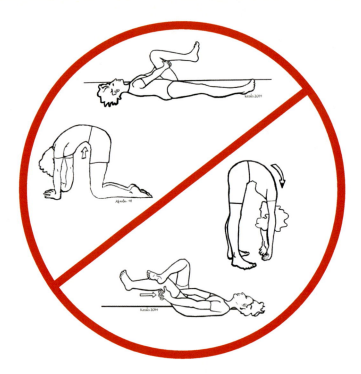

The stretches above shorten the muscles in front of the body. They may "feel good" because the muscles "want" to be short, but "feel good" does not always mean it is good. Shortening the muscles will increase your back pain in the long term.

While it is not possible to avoid bending or leaning forward occasionally, it is not a position you need to maintain for extended periods of time. Many tasks do not require it at all. You bend forward out of habit. You continue to take that position without even thinking about it. You just do it, even when you don't have to, but this constantly teaches the muscles to stay in that shortened position. Back pain results.

BACK PAIN

The examples of changes on page 5, and stretches on page 7, are given here to help you begin reversing the habits causing your back pain.

Simple Changes to End Chronic Pain presents pages of illustrated examples of sleeping, sitting, and standing postures that shorten the abdominal and hip muscles and result in back pain. It then gives practical suggestions for making the necessary changes, changes you can make at home.

Summary

All of this information may sound like just the opposite of what you have been told or read, or have learned about back pain. You are right – and that is what makes this book exciting.

What has been done to treat back pain, for the most part, has not worked. That is why it is at epidemic level and often the number one reason for missing work and changing how you live.

The main difference is that everyone has been looking at the structure of the back and spine, and basically treating symptoms. Patients experience recurring pain because the true cause has not been addressed..

The approach here is that back pain comes from muscles in the front of the body that have gotten tight or short. Because you continued to use them that way, they have learned to work from a tight position. There is nothing wrong with the muscles: no injury, strain, or damage. They are just doing what you have taught them to do. But that means when they get to a certain level of contraction, they will refer back pain. These referred pain patterns have been medically documented.

If you hurt when you walk, run, or play tennis, your doctor can run many tests and find nothing to explain your pain. If, however, you get evaluated by someone who runs or teaches tennis, they can tell you how you are using your muscles and body in a way that is causing imbalances and resulting in your pain. Make some simple changes, and life is good!

HIP PAIN

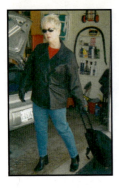 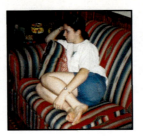 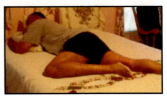

Hip-joint pain often comes from this muscle in the **low-back** area whose function is to twist the body and to bend it to one side.

Low Back

S H O R T

M U S C L E

P A I N

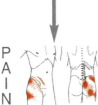

Hip Joint & Buttock

The postures shown above shorten this muscle on one side and pull it long on the other side. (Try the above postures and observe where tension occurs.)

When imbalanced and stressed by being in different positions on the right and left sides, the muscle will elicit or refer pain to the hip joint. The joint is fine, but because the referred pain is felt in the joint, the pain is usually diagnosed as bursitis or inflammation. Rest and medications are used as treatment. While this treatment may reduce the symptoms, the *muscle* remains short on one side and long on the other, and the pain continues in the hip joint.

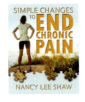 See a full explanation of muscle-referred pain in *Simple Changes to End Chronic Pain*.

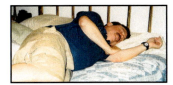

HIP PAIN

Teach the muscles to be balanced by sitting, standing, and sleeping with the body balanced on the right and left sides.

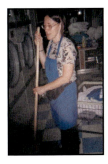 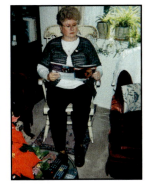

Then use stretch to teach a new muscle memory that allows the muscle to relax into an elongated position, resulting in pain-free movement.

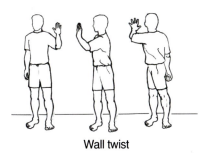
Wall twist

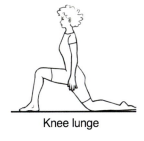
Knee lunge

 Suggestions for making these and other changes, and advice on all stretches that are the most helpful for hip-joint pain are included in *Simple Changes to End Chronic Pain.*

HIP PAIN

Additional Factors Contributing to Hip Pain

Stiff Shoes

Clip, clop! Shoes that don't bend can be a significant factor in straining the hip muscles that cause pain, particularly when walking. Stiff shoes change your walking motion, so you tend to walk flat-footed. If the foot in the shoe can't bend, ankle and knee movement are decreased. Then you have to lift or hike your hip to have room to bring your foot forward when taking a step. The bending of the foot as you walk, however, begins a smooth, even motion. Foot bends, ankle bends, knee bends: no hip hiking necessary to take a step and, therefore, no hip-joint pain.

Stiff, inflexible shoes are often recommended for plantar fasciitis. If the foot doesn't move, it may not hurt, but flexible or bendable shoes allow gentle movement, which is necessary if muscles are to learn to function without contraction.

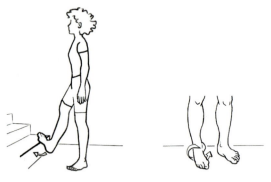

Calf step stretch   Ankle-foot roll

Shoe choices and a series of stretches associated with stiff shoes can be found in *Simple Changes to End Chronic Pain*.

HIP PAIN

Leg Length Inequality

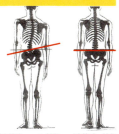
Without lift   With lift

A leg length inequality (LLI) can be observed, and should be evaluated, when one is standing. Check the line of the hips right and left, or notice a difference in your pants length.

A detailed description for determining LLI presence and correction is covered in detail in *Simple Changes to End Chronic Pain*.

The low-back and hip muscles pictured earlier are pulled long on the low leg side, and hiked or crunched on the longer leg side. Without correction, the imbalance of this muscle will result in hip-joint pain.

A suspecting indication of LLI may be kicking a leg out to one side when standing. While the body tries to adjust to this discrepancy, the muscle involved is still imbalanced and will refer pain to the hip joint.

Often, merely inserting a one quarter-inch heel lift in your shoe on the low side is enough to eliminate the muscle imbalances and the referred pain at the hip joint.

Stretches help teach the muscles involved to return to balanced, pain-free movement.

Crossover

It is important to make all the simple changes mentioned in posture, shoes, and leg length discrepancy, if pain is to be eliminated. It only takes one factor left unchanged to keep the muscle referring pain. The changes are yours to make.

SCIATICA PAIN

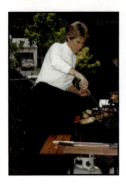
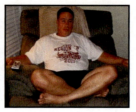
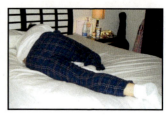

Hip

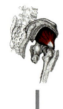

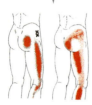

Buttock & Leg mimic "Sciatica"

"Sciatica" can be the result of the muscle shown here, which becomes involved because of the low back hip-pain muscle shown in the earlier section. The low-back muscle refers pain to the area of the hip joint where this "sciatica" muscle is situated. This results in the muscle beginning to refer its own pain down the back and side of the leg. In reality, it may be labeled "pseudo-sciatica," since it does not originate from the spinal disk, which is usually the diagnosis. Because the pain arises from incorrect muscle function, it is possible to eliminate it by changing how the muscle learns to work.

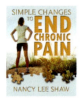

See the many postures that can be responsible for "pseudo-sciatica" in *Simple Changes to End Chronic Pain*. Suggestions for changing muscle patterns and stretches for muscle retraining are waiting for your attention.

SCIATICA PAIN

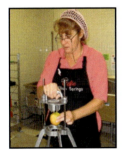
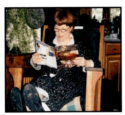
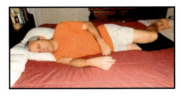

It is important to stand, sit, and sleep in an alignment that keeps the body even and balanced from right to left. Granted, it will take some specific focus for a few days to make correct movements and body positions a habit.

To teach the muscle to feel good in these new positions and to develop a memory, a habit, of staying balanced and elongated, you will need to perform a few stretches frequently.

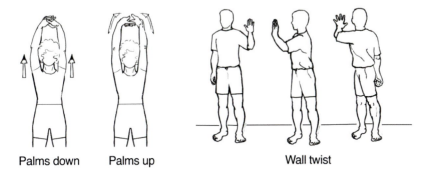

Palms down   Palms up   Wall twist

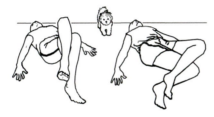

Crossover

SCIATICA PAIN

Summary

It may be new information to you that "sciatica," or "pseudo-sciatica," is the result of tight muscles, but the research and muscle pain referral patterns have been documented in the medical literature for over thirty years.

It takes a different way of evaluating and diagnosing the pain, and it takes time to devise a treatment plan. The main emphasis will be on identifying incorrect muscle function. There is nothing wrong with the muscles, other than they have been taught to work inefficiently and in pain-producing ways.

 Take the time to read and study the parent book, *Simple Changes to End Chronic Pain*, for an extensive explanation and plan devised for you to win the battle over chronic pain. It is exciting and sets you on a path of pain-free adventures.

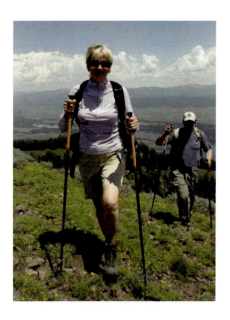

SCIATICA PAIN

Notes

Stress

Additional Factors Resulting in Muscle Shortness

Stress

Stress is a physical or psychological overload that elicits a tissue response. It is a normal part of life for everyone. Stress arises from things that are happening around you or to you on a regular basis, in your body, your mind, or your life.

The body is designed and expected to experience stress and to respond to it adequately. Stress becomes a negative factor when it is continuous and seemingly without end. Stress becomes "distress" that tenses the entire system, including the muscles. Muscles may already be tight from normal, everyday use and have not been stretched to a relaxed, balanced position. Add stress and muscles reach an increase level of tension, and begin to elicit pain that often includes back, hip, and "pseudo-sciatica" pain.

Several commonly experienced stress factors, besides the postures shown earlier, may activate abdominal, low back, and hip tension or tightness, resulting in associated back and hip pain:

- Lack of adequate sleep (7-8 hours), leading eventually to body fatigue. As muscles fatigue, they shorten as a protective way to be less vulnerable to strain or injury. Short muscle function results in a habitual pattern of being short and referring pain.

- Over-exercise, as in doing too many sit-ups or push-ups, or too many heavy resistance "curl-type" exercises such as bicep and chest exercises. It is important to work within a range that is comfortable for the muscles. This is especially true when you are in pain: stretching, not strengthening, is the desired way to eliminate the pain.

STRESS

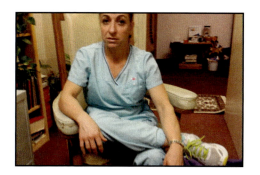

- Emotional tension that can lead to psychological strain. Pressure and stress may seem overwhelming, with no letup in sight. This stress may come from your job, or your family and friends. It may be from the past, today, or projected into the future. Whichever, your overactivated nervous system tightens muscles that can result in referred back, hip, and "sciatica" pain.
- Cold exposure tightens muscles, making it difficult to relax and elongate them.
- Continual coughing causes muscle contraction and pain.

The chronic pain you experience can result from viewing your life as a series of unrelenting stresses.

Follow stress reduction practices that will shut off your mind to constant worry, frustration, anger, hurt, and anxiety. Forgiveness is a powerful tool. It may seem easier said than done, but if you are willing to make time to participate in some of the following practices, it will make a difference and lead you toward more active, pain-free adventures.

STRESS

Take time:
- To eat breakfast.
- To look around when you walk out the door and enjoy the beauty of the outdoors.
- To put aside your electronics on the way to work and listen to music.
- If something is unsettling or upsetting, to deal with it at once by addressing it in the open, not in the silence of your mind.
- To add "get up and move" moments every two hours throughout your day.
- To eat lunch away from your desk.
- To be reasonable about when you end your work day.
- To give up your electronics at home, and enjoy your family and friends instead.
- To avoid going to bed without having done something fun at some point during the day or evening.

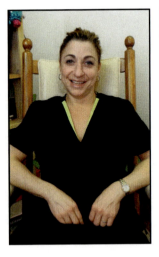

Smile, this life really is a good life. Do your part in making it good.

Notes

NUTRITION

Nutrition

"Oh, no! On top of everything else, I am supposed to eat breakfast, lunch, and dinner, and have snacks in between. And it is supposed to be healthy food as well."

True, but it doesn't have to be such a difficult thing to do. It is often thought that keeping muscles healthy is more than a 50 percent nutritional factor. It is important, but doable.

While nutrition should be a healthy balance of protein, carbohydrates, and fats, remember that muscles need protein to function, and more importantly, they need protein to repair. But balance is important.

Here are a few suggestions:
- Do not skip any meals.
- Focus on some protein for breakfast: hardboiled or scrambled egg, or toast with peanut or almond butter.
- Snack on seeds and nuts.
- Have fruit and veggies with your lunch.
- A bigger lunch than dinner is desirable.
- Snack again on fruit, yogurt (plain with your own nuts or fruit).
- No sodas, candy, or cookies.
- A light dinner best eaten by 7 p.m.
- Do not avoid fats. Salmon, trout, catfish, avocados, mixed nuts, olive oil, coconut oil, nut butters, and walnuts are all healthy fats. Occasional beef and pork are acceptable also.

Not just coffee and danish

Just a couple of primary key points:
- Do not skip meals.
- Do not start your day or snack on sugary foods.

NUTRITION

Okay, let's get to "what are some good recipes" you can make. Below are some recipes that are easy to prepare, can be made for one person or many, store easily and even taste good.

Egg Breakfast

This recipe can easily be prepared ahead of time, even the night before. Keep in the refrigerator until you are ready to bake.

Grease a 9x13–inch baking pan (smaller if you make half a recipe.)

Ingredients:
4 cups croutons or cubed bread
1-½ cups cheddar (or preference) *cheese* (reduce to your taste)
Combine these two ingredients. Place on the bottom of the pan.

8 eggs (remember you can easily made half a recipe – 4 eggs)
4 cups milk
1 teaspoon salt
1 teaspoon mustard
1-¼ teaspoons minced onion or ½ teaspoon onion salt
Mix and pour this mixture over the croutons and cheese.
(Optional: you may add mushrooms, bacon pieces, peppers, etc.)

Bake at 325 degrees F. for 1 hour (less if smaller recipe).
To test if it is fully cooked, make a cut in the center of the dish. The knife should come out clean: no stickiness.

(Gail R., Illinois)

NUTRITION

Potato Pancakes

This recipe is good for breakfast, lunch, or even dinner. Not a bad snack either.

Ingredients:
3–4 potatoes (number depends on how many pancakes you want. You will probably get 3 pancakes from each medium potato.)
1 egg per potato (this helps it all stick together)
2 tablespoons flour
1 teaspoon salt
¼ teaspoon pepper
Veggies-pick your favorites:
  1 cup carrot
  1-½ zucchini
  1 teaspoon onion
  ½ cup green/red pepper
  ½ cup mushrooms

Grate the potatoes then blot with a paper towel as they will be a little watery.

Beat together egg, flour, salt, and pepper.

Grate vegetables and cut up mushrooms and peppers.
Mix and stir the potatoes and vegetables into the egg mixture.

Drop by spoonfuls onto a nonstick or oil-sprayed baking pan (cookie sheet or similar). Flatten slightly.

Bake at 425 degrees F. for 8–15 minutes until bottom of pancake is brown. Flip or turn over and bake an additional 10 minutes.

(Family Favorite, Nebraska)

NUTRITION

Banana Blueberry Muffins

This is an easy recipe that serves well for breakfast or a snack.

Ingredients:
2 extra-ripe medium bananas, peeled
2 eggs
¼ cup brown sugar, molasses, or honey
½ cup butter, melted
1 cup blueberries
1 teaspoon vanilla
2-¼ cups flour
2 teaspoons baking powder
½ teaspoon ground cinnamon
½ teaspoon salt
(Optional: ½ cup whole or chopped walnuts or pecans)

Mash bananas.

In medium bowl, combine bananas, eggs, sugar, and butter until well blended.

Stir in blueberries and vanilla.

In large bowl, combine flour, baking powder, cinnamon and salt.

Stir banana mixture into flour mixture until evenly moistened. Add nuts if desired.

Spoon batter into greased muffin tin cups.

Bake at 350 degrees F. for 25–30 minutes or until wooden pick inserted in the center comes out clean.

(Modified from *The Muffin Cookbook*, Crescent Books, 1990.)

NUTRITION

Peanut Butter Banana Muffins

This is a great snack muffin.

Ingredients:
1-½ cups flour
1 teaspoon baking powder
1 teaspoon baking soda
½ cup yogurt
½ cup butter, melted
½ cup chunky peanut or almond butter
¼ cup sugar, molasses, or honey
2 ripe bananas, mashed
1 egg
1 teaspoon vanilla

In small bowl, combine flour, baking powder, and baking soda.

In large bowl, beat yogurt, butter, peanut or almond butter, and sugar, molasses or honey.

Add bananas, egg, and vanilla to large bowl; mix well.

Add flour mixture and stir until moistened.

Fill paper-lined or greased muffin cups ¾ full.
(Optional: top with chopped nuts)

Bake at 350 degrees F. for 25–30 minutes or until wooden pick inserted in the center comes out clean.

(Modified from *The Muffin Cookbook*, Crescent Books, 1990.)

NUTRITION

Burger Special

Ingredients:

1 lb. hamburger (ground turkey or pork can also be used)
1 package of your favorite dry soup mix
1 egg
¼ cup bread crumbs or cooked rice
1 tablespoon Worchester Shire sauce or BBQ sauce
Optional: sautéed onions, mushrooms, green/red peppers or other favorites

This is an easy recipe to make your own version.

Place all ingredients in large bowl and mix—easiest to mix with hands.

Depending on the size of burger you want, make a ball of some of the mixture and place in a greased pan or skillet. Flatten the patty to desired thickness.

Cook about 5–6 minutes, flip over and cook another 5–6 minutes. Mmmm good!

These burger patties can be made up, flattened and placed in the freezer for future use. Handy for a quick meal.

Virginia

NUTRITION

Summary

You do not have to live with chronic pain! Let me say that again, you do not have to live with chronic pain!

This supplement, Back and Hip Pain, is designed to start you on the path to pain-free living. An expanded version of the information can be found in *Simple Changes to End Chronic Pain*.

I know many of you have tried a number of traditional approaches to dealing with back and hip pain. It hasn't work, at least not to the point of really ending the pain. Now you have an explanation for the pain and you have simple changes that you can practice right at home that will eliminate your pain.

It will seem too easy. It is not, it just works. You owe it to yourself to try it. You have nothing to lose, and a pain-free living adventure to gain.

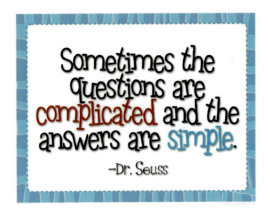

Notes

Made in the USA
Middletown, DE
08 August 2020